Non-Starch Vegetables Guide for Beginners

Importance of Non-Starch Vegetables in Diet

By

Leith Glendon

Copyright@2024

Table of Contents

CHAPTER 1

Introduction to Non-Starch Vegetables

1.1 What are Non-Starch Vegetables

Non-starch vegetables, often referred to simply as vegetables, encompass a broad array of plant-based foods that are characterized by their low starch content. These vegetables are a vital component of a balanced diet and are distinguished from starchy vegetables primarily by their carbohydrate composition. While starchy vegetables such as potatoes, corn, and peas contain higher levels of carbohydrates in the form of starch, non-starch vegetables have relatively lower amounts of starch and are typically richer in fiber, vitamins, minerals, and phytonutrients.

Non-starch vegetables come in a diverse range of shapes, sizes, colors, and flavors, reflecting the immense variety found in the plant kingdom. They include leafy greens like spinach, kale, and lettuce; cruciferous vegetables such as broccoli, cauliflower, and Brussels sprouts; root vegetables like carrots, beets, and turnips; allium vegetables including onions, garlic, and leeks; nightshade vegetables such as tomatoes, eggplants, and peppers; and an assortment of other vegetables like cucumber, zucchini, and mushrooms.

These vegetables are prized for their nutritional density and are renowned for their ability to contribute to overall health and well-being. They are typically low in calories and fat while being rich sources of essential nutrients like vitamins A, C, and K, as well as minerals like potassium, magnesium, and folate. Moreover, non-starch vegetables are packed with dietary fiber, which supports digestive health, promotes satiety, and helps regulate blood sugar levels.

Beyond their nutritional value, non-starch vegetables are celebrated for their versatility in the culinary world. They serve as the foundation for countless recipes, from hearty salads and stir-fries to soups, stews, and side dishes. Their vibrant colors, textures, and flavors enhance the sensory experience of meals, making them both visually appealing and delicious. non-starch vegetables lend themselves to various cooking techniques, including steaming, roasting, grilling, and sautéing, allowing for endless creativity in the kitchen.

In addition to their culinary appeal, non-starch vegetables play a crucial role in promoting environmental sustainability and reducing the carbon footprint of food production. Compared to animal-based foods, the cultivation of vegetables generally requires fewer natural resources like water and land and produces fewer greenhouse gas emissions. Therefore, incorporating more non-starch vegetables into one's diet can contribute to more sustainable food systems and mitigate the environmental impact of food consumption.

non-starch vegetables represent a cornerstone of a nutritious and sustainable diet. By incorporating an abundant variety of these plant-based foods into daily meals, individuals can reap a multitude of health benefits while enjoying the diverse flavors and textures that nature has to offer. Whether consumed raw or cooked, as a main dish or a side, non-starch vegetables are indispensable for promoting health, culinary creativity, and environmental stewardship.

1.2 Importance of Non-Starch Vegetables in Diet

The importance of non-starch vegetables in the diet cannot be overstated, as they offer a plethora of health benefits that contribute to overall well-being. Here are some key reasons why non-starch vegetables are essential components of a balanced diet:

1. Nutrient Density: Non-starch vegetables are nutrient powerhouses, packed with vitamins, minerals, and phytonutrients essential for optimal health. They are particularly rich in vitamins A, C, and K, as well as folate, potassium, magnesium, and

antioxidants. These nutrients play vital roles in various bodily functions, including immune function, bone health, cardiovascular health, and skin health.

2. Fiber Content: Non-starch vegetables are high in dietary fiber, which is crucial for digestive health and regular bowel movements. Fiber helps prevent constipation, promotes satiety, and regulates blood sugar levels, which can aid in weight management and reduce the risk of developing chronic diseases such as type 2 diabetes and heart disease.

3. Low in Calories and Fat: Non-starch vegetables are naturally low in calories and fat, making them ideal for those looking to maintain or lose weight. They provide bulk and volume to meals without adding excess calories, allowing individuals to feel satisfied while consuming fewer overall calories. Additionally, their low fat content makes them heart-healthy choices that can help

lower cholesterol levels and reduce the risk of cardiovascular disease.

4. Disease Prevention: The consumption of non-starch vegetables has been associated with a lower risk of various chronic diseases, including certain types of cancer, such as lung, colorectal, and prostate cancer. The antioxidants and phytochemicals found in non-starch vegetables have been shown to neutralize harmful free radicals in the body, thereby reducing oxidative stress and inflammation, which are underlying factors in the development of chronic diseases.

5. Blood Sugar Control: Non-starch vegetables have a low glycemic index, meaning they have minimal impact on blood sugar levels when consumed. This makes them suitable choices for individuals with diabetes or those at risk of developing diabetes, as they can help stabilize blood sugar levels and improve insulin sensitivity.

6. Hydration and Detoxification: Many non-starch vegetables have high water content, which can contribute to hydration and promote healthy skin and kidney function. Additionally, certain vegetables like leafy greens and cruciferous vegetables contain compounds that support the body's natural detoxification processes, helping to eliminate toxins and waste products from the body.

7. Versatility and Culinary Enjoyment: Non-starch vegetables come in a wide variety of flavors, textures, and colors, making them versatile ingredients that can be incorporated into a myriad of dishes. From salads and stir-fries to soups, stews, and side dishes, the culinary possibilities are endless. Experimenting with different types of non-starch vegetables can add excitement and variety to meals, making healthy eating enjoyable and sustainable in the long term.

non-starch vegetables are essential components of a healthy diet, offering an array of nutrients, fiber, and health-promoting compounds that support overall health and well-being. By including a diverse selection of non-starch vegetables in daily meals, individuals can enhance their nutritional intake, reduce the risk of chronic diseases, and enjoy delicious, satisfying meals that nourish the body and soul.

1.3 Nutritional Value of Non-Starch Vegetables

Understanding the nutritional value of non-starch vegetables is crucial for making informed dietary choices and optimizing health. Non-starch vegetables are rich in essential nutrients, dietary fiber, and phytochemicals, all of which contribute to their nutritional profile and health-promoting properties. Here's an overview of the nutritional value of non-starch vegetables:

1. **Vitamins**: Non-starch vegetables are excellent sources of various vitamins, including:

    - Vitamin A: Crucial for vision health, immune function, and skin health.

    - Vitamin C: An antioxidant that supports immune function, collagen synthesis, and wound healing.

    - Vitamin K: Essential for blood clotting and bone health.

    - B vitamins (e.g., folate, riboflavin, niacin): Important for energy metabolism, red blood cell production, and nervous system function.

2. **Minerals**: Non-starch vegetables provide an array of minerals necessary for various physiological functions, such as:

- Potassium: Important for heart health, blood pressure regulation, and muscle function.

- Magnesium: Involved in over 300 enzymatic reactions in the body, including energy production and muscle function.

- Calcium: Critical for bone health and muscle function.

- Iron: Necessary for oxygen transport in the blood and energy metabolism.

3. **Dietary Fiber**: Non-starch vegetables are high in dietary fiber, which offers numerous health benefits, including:

    - Digestive health: Fiber promotes regular bowel movements, prevents constipation, and supports a healthy gut microbiome.

- Weight management: Fiber adds bulk to meals, promoting feelings of fullness and reducing overall calorie intake.

- Blood sugar control: Fiber slows down the absorption of glucose, helping to stabilize blood sugar levels and improve insulin sensitivity.

- Heart health: Soluble fiber can help lower cholesterol levels, reducing the risk of heart disease.

4. **Phytochemicals and Antioxidants**: Non-starch vegetables contain various phytochemicals, such as flavonoids, carotenoids, and polyphenols, which have antioxidant and anti-inflammatory properties. These compounds help protect cells from damage caused by free radicals, reduce inflammation, and may lower the risk of chronic diseases,

including cancer and cardiovascular disease.

5.   **Water Content**: Many non-starch vegetables have high water content, contributing to hydration and supporting overall health. Proper hydration is essential for maintaining bodily functions, regulating body temperature, and promoting healthy skin.

6.   **Low in Calories and Fat**: Non-starch vegetables are naturally low in calories and fat, making them ideal for weight management and overall health. They provide essential nutrients and volume to meals without adding excess calories or unhealthy fats.

non-starch vegetables are nutritional powerhouses, providing a wide range of vitamins, minerals, fiber, and phytochemicals essential for optimal health. Including a variety of non-starch vegetables in your diet can help ensure adequate nutrient intake, promote digestive health, support weight management, and reduce the risk of chronic diseases.

CHAPTER 2

Types of Non-Starch Vegetables

2.1 Leafy Greens

Leafy greens are a diverse group of non-starch vegetables characterized by their tender, edible leaves. They are prized for their vibrant colors, distinctive flavors, and impressive nutritional profiles. Here are some common types of leafy greens:

1. **Spinach**: Spinach is a nutrient-rich leafy green known for its mild flavor and versatility. It is an excellent source of vitamins A, C, and K, as well as folate, iron, and antioxidants. Spinach can be eaten raw in salads, sautéed as a side dish, or incorporated into soups, smoothies, and pasta dishes.

2. **Kale**: Kale is often hailed as a superfood due to its exceptional

nutritional content. It is rich in vitamins A, C, and K, as well as calcium, potassium, and antioxidants like lutein and zeaxanthin. Kale has a slightly bitter taste and a hearty texture, making it ideal for salads, stir-fries, soups, and smoothies.

3. **Lettuce**: Lettuce encompasses various types, including iceberg, romaine, butterhead, and leaf lettuce. These greens are low in calories and provide vitamins A, C, and K, as well as folate and potassium. Lettuce is commonly used as a base for salads, sandwiches, and wraps, adding crunch and freshness to dishes.

4. **Arugula**: Arugula, also known as rocket, has a peppery flavor and tender leaves. It is rich in vitamins A, C, and K, as well as folate, calcium, and potassium. Arugula adds a zesty kick to salads, sandwiches, pizzas, and pasta dishes.

5. **Swiss Chard**: Swiss chard features colorful stems and dark green leaves with a slightly earthy taste. It is a good source of vitamins A, C, and K, as well as magnesium, potassium, and fiber. Swiss chard can be sautéed, steamed, or added to soups, stews, and casseroles.

6. **Collard Greens**: Collard greens have thick, sturdy leaves and a slightly bitter flavor. They are packed with vitamins A, C, and K, as well as calcium, folate, and fiber. Collard greens are often braised, steamed, or added to soups and stews, especially in Southern cuisine.

7. **Bok Choy**: Bok choy, also known as Chinese cabbage, has crisp, white stems and dark green leaves. It is rich in vitamins A, C, and K, as well as calcium, potassium, and antioxidants. Bok choy is commonly used in Asian stir-fries, soups, and noodle dishes.

8. **Watercress**: Watercress has a peppery taste and delicate leaves. It is loaded with vitamins A, C, and K, as well as calcium, iron, and antioxidants. Watercress adds a bold flavor to salads, sandwiches, and soups, and is often used as a garnish.

These are just a few examples of the diverse array of leafy greens available. Including a variety of leafy greens in your diet can provide an abundance of nutrients and contribute to overall health and well-being.

2.2 Cruciferous Vegetables

Cruciferous vegetables belong to the Brassicaceae family and are characterized by their cross-shaped flowers. They are renowned for their distinctive flavors, crunchy textures, and numerous health benefits. Here are some common types of cruciferous vegetables:

1. **Broccoli**: Broccoli is a nutrient-dense vegetable packed with vitamins C and K, folate, fiber, and

antioxidants such as sulforaphane. It has a distinctive green color and can be enjoyed steamed, roasted, stir-fried, or raw in salads and crudité platters.

2. **Cauliflower**: Cauliflower is versatile and can be cooked in various ways, including roasting, steaming, or mashed as a low-carb alternative to mashed potatoes. It is rich in vitamin C, vitamin K, folate, fiber, and antioxidants like glucosinolates.

3. **Cabbage**: Cabbage comes in different varieties such as green, red, and Savoy. It is a good source of vitamins C and K, as well as fiber and antioxidants. Cabbage can be shredded and used in salads, fermented to make sauerkraut, or cooked in stir-fries, soups, and stews.

4. **Brussels Sprouts**: Brussels sprouts are small, leafy green vegetables that resemble miniature cabbages. They are packed with vitamins C and K, as well as fiber, folate, and

antioxidants. Brussels sprouts can be roasted, sautéed, or steamed as a delicious side dish.

5. **Kale**: Kale, while also a leafy green, is often grouped with cruciferous vegetables due to its nutritional profile. It is rich in vitamins A, C, and K, as well as calcium, potassium, and antioxidants. Kale can be enjoyed raw in salads, sautéed, or added to soups and smoothies.

6. **Arugula**: Arugula has a peppery flavor and is commonly used in salads and sandwiches. It is rich in vitamins A, C, and K, as well as calcium and antioxidants. Arugula adds a unique flavor and texture to dishes and pairs well with various ingredients.

2.3 Root Vegetables

Root vegetables are plant roots that are harvested for culinary use. They come in a variety of shapes, sizes, and colors and are prized for their earthy flavors and nutrient-rich profiles. Here are some common types of root vegetables:

1. **Carrots**: Carrots are known for their vibrant orange color and sweet flavor. They are rich in beta-carotene, which is converted into vitamin A in the body, as well as vitamins C and K, fiber, and potassium. Carrots can be eaten raw as a snack, roasted, steamed, or added to soups and stews.

2. **Potatoes**: Potatoes are one of the most versatile root vegetables and come in various types such as russet, red, and Yukon Gold. They are a good source of carbohydrates, potassium, vitamin C, and fiber. Potatoes can be boiled, baked, mashed, or fried and are used in numerous dishes worldwide.

3. **Sweet Potatoes**: Sweet potatoes have a naturally sweet flavor and are rich in beta-carotene, vitamins A and

C, fiber, and antioxidants. They can be baked, roasted, mashed, or used in desserts like pies and cakes.

4. **Beets**: Beets have a deep red color and a sweet, earthy flavor. They are rich in vitamins C and B6, folate, manganese, and antioxidants like betalains. Beets can be roasted, boiled, grated raw into salads, or pickled.

5. **Turnips**: Turnips have a slightly peppery flavor and can be eaten raw or cooked. They are a good source of vitamins C and K, as well as fiber and antioxidants. Turnips can be roasted, mashed, or added to soups and stews.

6. **Radishes**: Radishes come in various colors and have a crisp texture and peppery flavor. They are low in calories and a good source of vitamin C, fiber, and antioxidants. Radishes can be eaten raw in salads, pickled, or roasted.

Incorporating both cruciferous and root vegetables into your diet can provide a wide range of nutrients and contribute to overall health and culinary enjoyment.

2.4 Allium Vegetables

Allium vegetables belong to the Allium genus and are characterized by their pungent aroma and distinctive flavors. They are widely used in cooking to add depth and complexity to dishes. Here are some common types of allium vegetables:

1. **Onions**: Onions come in various colors and sizes, including white, yellow, and red onions. They have a sharp, pungent flavor when raw, which mellows and sweetens when cooked. Onions are rich in antioxidants, particularly quercetin, as well as vitamin C, fiber, and prebiotics that promote gut health. They are versatile ingredients used in soups, stews, sauces, stir-fries, and salads.

2. **Garlic**: Garlic is renowned for its strong flavor and aroma and is used in cuisines worldwide. It contains sulfur compounds like allicin, which have antimicrobial and immune-boosting properties. Garlic is also rich in antioxidants, vitamins C and B6, and minerals like manganese and selenium. It is used fresh, minced, or crushed in a wide range of savory dishes, sauces, marinades, and dressings.

3. **Shallots**: Shallots are small, bulbous vegetables with a milder flavor than onions and garlic. They have a slightly sweet and delicate taste and are often used in French and Asian cuisines. Shallots contain antioxidants, vitamins A and C, and minerals like potassium and manganese. They are commonly used in sauces, vinaigrettes, and as a flavoring agent in various dishes.

4. **Leeks**: Leeks have a mild onion flavor and a unique cylindrical shape with layers of white and green parts.

They are rich in vitamins A, K, and folate, as well as antioxidants like polyphenols and flavonoids. Leeks are versatile vegetables used in soups, stews, quiches, and as a flavorful addition to sautéed dishes.

5. **Scallions (Green Onions)**: Scallions have a mild onion flavor and are prized for their crisp texture and vibrant green color. They are rich in vitamins K and C, as well as antioxidants like flavonoids and carotenoids. Scallions are commonly used as a garnish in salads, soups, stir-fries, and noodle dishes.

6. **Chives**: Chives have a mild onion flavor with a hint of garlic and are often used as a garnish or flavoring herb. They are rich in vitamins A and C, as well as minerals like calcium and potassium. Chives are commonly used to enhance the flavor of dishes like baked potatoes, omelets, salads, and soups.

Allium vegetables not only add flavor and depth to dishes but also offer numerous health benefits due to their rich nutrient and antioxidant content. Including a variety of allium vegetables in your diet can promote overall health and culinary enjoyment.

2.5 Nightshade Vegetables

Nightshade vegetables belong to the Solanaceae family and include a variety of plants known for their edible fruits, which are often used as vegetables in cooking. Despite their popularity, some people may be sensitive to certain compounds found in nightshade vegetables, particularly solanine and glycoalkaloids, which can cause adverse reactions in sensitive individuals. However, for most people, nightshade vegetables are nutritious and offer a range of health benefits. Here are some common types of nightshade vegetables:

1. **Tomatoes**: Tomatoes are one of the most widely consumed nightshade vegetables and are prized for their

juicy texture and tangy flavor. They are rich in vitamins A and C, as well as antioxidants like lycopene, which has been linked to a reduced risk of certain cancers and heart disease. Tomatoes are used in numerous dishes, including sauces, salads, soups, and sandwiches.

2. **Bell Peppers**: Bell peppers come in various colors, including red, yellow, orange, and green, and are known for their sweet flavor and crunchy texture. They are rich in vitamins A and C, as well as antioxidants like beta-carotene and quercetin. Bell peppers can be eaten raw in salads, stuffed, roasted, or added to stir-fries, fajitas, and kebabs.

3. **Eggplants**: Eggplants have a rich, meaty texture and a slightly bitter taste. They are a good source of dietary fiber, vitamins C and K, and antioxidants like nasunin, which may help protect cells from damage. Eggplants are used in various cuisines worldwide, including

Mediterranean, Middle Eastern, and
Asian dishes, such as eggplant
parmesan, moussaka, and baba
ganoush.

4. **Potatoes**: Potatoes are versatile tuber
   vegetables that come in different
   varieties, including russet, red,
   Yukon Gold, and fingerling potatoes.
   They are rich in carbohydrates,
   potassium, and vitamin C, as well as
   fiber, especially when consumed
   with the skin. Potatoes can be boiled,
   baked, mashed, or fried and are used
   in numerous dishes like mashed
   potatoes, French fries, and potato
   salad.

5. **Chili Peppers**: Chili peppers,
   including varieties like jalapeños,
   habaneros, and serranos, are known
   for their spicy heat and are used to
   add flavor and heat to dishes. They
   contain capsaicin, a compound that
   has been shown to have anti-
   inflammatory and pain-relieving
   properties. Chili peppers are used in

salsas, hot sauces, curries, and spicy dishes around the world.

6. **Tomatillos**: Tomatillos are small, green, tart fruits encased in papery husks and are commonly used in Mexican cuisine. They are rich in vitamins C and K, as well as antioxidants like quercetin. Tomatillos are used to make salsa verde, sauces, and soups, adding a tangy flavor to dishes.

Despite their potential for sensitivity in some individuals, nightshade vegetables offer a range of nutrients and culinary versatility. Including a variety of nightshade vegetables in your diet can provide essential vitamins, minerals, and antioxidants while adding flavor and diversity to meals.

2.6 Other Non-Starch Vegetables

Beyond leafy greens, cruciferous vegetables, root vegetables, allium vegetables, and nightshade vegetables, there is a vast array of other non-starch vegetables that offer unique flavors, textures, and nutritional profiles. Here are some examples of other non-starch vegetables:

1. **Cucumbers**: Cucumbers are crisp, refreshing vegetables with a high water content. They are low in calories and rich in vitamins K and C, as well as antioxidants like cucurbitacins and flavonoids. Cucumbers are commonly enjoyed raw in salads, sandwiches, and pickles.

2. **Zucchini**: Zucchini, also known as courgette, is a versatile summer squash with a mild flavor and tender texture. It is low in calories and carbohydrates and rich in vitamins C and B6, potassium, and antioxidants. Zucchini can be grilled, sautéed, roasted, or spiralized into noodles as a low-carb pasta alternative.

3. **Mushrooms**: Mushrooms are fungi that are often considered vegetables

in culinary terms. They come in various types, including button, cremini, portobello, shiitake, and oyster mushrooms, each with its own flavor and texture. Mushrooms are low in calories and rich in protein, fiber, vitamins B and D, and minerals like selenium and potassium. They are used in a wide range of dishes, including soups, stir-fries, sauces, and risottos.

4. **Peas**: Peas are small, round green vegetables that belong to the legume family. They are rich in vitamins A, C, and K, as well as fiber, protein, and antioxidants like flavonoids and carotenoids. Peas can be eaten fresh or frozen and are used in dishes like soups, salads, stir-fries, and risottos.

5. **Celery**: Celery is a crunchy, fibrous vegetable with a mild, slightly bitter flavor. It is low in calories and rich in vitamins A, K, and C, as well as minerals like potassium and folate. Celery is commonly used as a snack,

in salads, soups, stews, and as a flavoring agent in stocks and sauces.

6. **Asparagus**: Asparagus is a tender, spear-like vegetable with a unique flavor and texture. It is rich in vitamins A, C, and K, as well as folate, fiber, and antioxidants like glutathione. Asparagus can be steamed, grilled, roasted, or sautéed and is often enjoyed as a side dish or added to salads, omelets, and pasta dishes.

7. **Artichokes**: Artichokes are thistle-like vegetables prized for their tender hearts and meaty leaves. They are rich in fiber, vitamins C and K, folate, and antioxidants like cynarin and silymarin. Artichokes can be steamed, boiled, roasted, or grilled and are commonly served with dips or added to salads, pizzas, and pasta dishes.

These are just a few examples of the many other non-starch vegetables available. Including a variety of non-starch vegetables in your diet can provide a wide range of nutrients and culinary enjoyment while promoting overall health and well-being.

CHAPTER 3

Health Benefits of Non-Starch Vegetables

3.1 Rich Source of Vitamins and Minerals

Non-starch vegetables are prized for their abundance of vitamins and minerals, making them essential components of a healthy diet. Here are some key health benefits associated with the rich vitamins and minerals found in non-starch vegetables:

1. **Vitamin A**: Many non-starch vegetables, particularly those with vibrant colors like carrots, sweet potatoes, and spinach, are rich sources of beta-carotene, a precursor to vitamin A. Vitamin A is essential for vision health, immune function, and skin health. It supports the proper functioning of the eyes, helps maintain a healthy immune system,

and promotes the growth and repair of skin tissues.

2. **Vitamin C**: Non-starch vegetables such as bell peppers, broccoli, and kale are excellent sources of vitamin C, a powerful antioxidant that plays a crucial role in immune function, collagen synthesis, and wound healing. Vitamin C helps protect cells from damage caused by free radicals, supports the immune system's response to infections, and promotes the absorption of iron from plant-based foods.

3. **Vitamin K**: Leafy greens like kale, spinach, and Swiss chard are rich in vitamin K, which is essential for blood clotting and bone health. Vitamin K helps regulate blood clotting by facilitating the production of proteins necessary for the clotting process. Additionally, vitamin K plays a role in bone metabolism and may help reduce the risk of fractures and osteoporosis.

4. **Folate (Vitamin B9)**: Non-starch vegetables such as asparagus, broccoli, and Brussels sprouts are sources of folate, a B vitamin important for DNA synthesis and cell division. Folate is particularly important during pregnancy as it helps prevent neural tube defects in the developing fetus. It also supports red blood cell production and helps maintain cardiovascular health.

5. **Potassium**: Many non-starch vegetables, including potatoes, sweet potatoes, and spinach, are rich sources of potassium, an essential mineral that plays a key role in fluid balance, muscle function, and blood pressure regulation. Potassium helps counteract the effects of sodium in the body, promoting healthy blood pressure levels and reducing the risk of hypertension and cardiovascular disease.

6. **Magnesium**: Leafy greens, legumes, and nuts are sources of magnesium, a mineral involved in over 300

enzymatic reactions in the body. Magnesium supports muscle and nerve function, regulates blood sugar levels, and contributes to bone health. Adequate magnesium intake may also reduce the risk of type 2 diabetes and improve mood and sleep quality.

7. **Iron**: Non-starch vegetables such as spinach, kale, and lentils are sources of non-heme iron, the type of iron found in plant-based foods. While non-heme iron is not as easily absorbed as heme iron from animal sources, consuming vitamin C-rich foods alongside non-heme iron can enhance its absorption. Iron is essential for oxygen transport in the blood and energy metabolism.

Incorporating a variety of non-starch vegetables into your diet can provide a wide range of vitamins and minerals essential for overall health and well-being. Whether eaten raw or cooked, these nutrient-dense foods contribute to a balanced diet and support optimal health.

3.2 High in Dietary Fiber

Non-starch vegetables are known for their high fiber content, which offers numerous health benefits. Here's why the high dietary fiber content in non-starch vegetables is advantageous:

1. **Promotes Digestive Health**: Dietary fiber adds bulk to stool, softening it and promoting regular bowel movements. This helps prevent constipation and reduces the risk of developing hemorrhoids and other digestive issues. Fiber also contributes to the overall health of the digestive tract by supporting the growth of beneficial gut bacteria and maintaining a healthy gut microbiome.

2. **Supports Weight Management**: Foods high in dietary fiber are often low in calories and can help promote feelings of fullness and satiety. By increasing meal volume without adding extra calories, fiber-rich non-starch vegetables can help control

appetite and reduce overall calorie intake, making them valuable for weight management and weight loss efforts.

3. **Stabilizes Blood Sugar Levels**: High-fiber foods, including non-starch vegetables, can help stabilize blood sugar levels by slowing down the absorption of sugars from the digestive tract. This can help prevent spikes and crashes in blood sugar levels, making fiber-rich foods particularly beneficial for individuals with diabetes or those at risk of developing the condition.

4. **Lowers Cholesterol Levels**: Soluble fiber, found in foods like beans, lentils, and certain non-starch vegetables like Brussels sprouts and eggplant, has been shown to help lower LDL (bad) cholesterol levels in the blood. By binding to cholesterol and bile acids in the digestive tract, soluble fiber helps remove them from the body,

reducing the risk of heart disease and stroke.

5. **Improves Gut Health**: Dietary fiber serves as a prebiotic, providing fuel for beneficial bacteria in the gut. By promoting the growth of these beneficial bacteria, fiber helps maintain a healthy balance of gut microbiota, which is essential for immune function, nutrient absorption, and overall gut health. A healthy gut microbiome has been linked to numerous health benefits, including reduced inflammation and improved mental health.

6. **Reduces the Risk of Chronic Diseases**: Consuming a diet high in fiber-rich foods, including non-starch vegetables, has been associated with a reduced risk of developing chronic diseases such as heart disease, type 2 diabetes, and certain types of cancer. The protective effects of dietary fiber are thought to be mediated through its effects on digestion, metabolism, and inflammation.

7. **Aids in Weight Management**:
    Fiber-rich foods are typically low in
    energy density, meaning they
    provide fewer calories per gram
    compared to foods high in fat and
    sugar. This makes non-starch
    vegetables an excellent choice for
    weight management, as they can help
    increase satiety while providing
    essential nutrients and promoting
    overall health.

A variety of fiber-rich non-starch vegetables into your diet can help support digestive health, regulate blood sugar levels, lower cholesterol, and reduce the risk of chronic diseases. Aim to include a colorful assortment of vegetables in your meals to maximize their fiber content and reap the numerous health benefits they offer.

3.3 Antioxidant Properties

Non-starch vegetables are rich in antioxidants, compounds that help neutralize harmful free radicals in the body. Here's how the antioxidant properties of non-starch vegetables benefit health:

1. **Protect Against Cellular Damage**: Antioxidants in non-starch vegetables, such as vitamins A, C, and E, as well as phytochemicals like flavonoids and carotenoids, help protect cells from oxidative damage caused by free radicals. This reduces the risk of chronic diseases such as cancer, heart disease, and neurodegenerative disorders.

2. **Support Immune Function**: Antioxidants play a crucial role in supporting the immune system by neutralizing free radicals that can damage immune cells. By reducing oxidative stress and inflammation, antioxidants help enhance immune function and improve the body's ability to fight off infections and illnesses.

3. **Promote Skin Health**: Antioxidants like vitamin C and beta-carotene contribute to healthy skin by

protecting against UV-induced damage, reducing inflammation, and promoting collagen synthesis. Including antioxidant-rich non-starch vegetables in the diet can help maintain youthful skin, prevent premature aging, and protect against skin conditions like wrinkles and sunburn.

4. **Reduce Inflammation**: Chronic inflammation is a contributing factor to many diseases, including arthritis, cardiovascular disease, and autoimmune disorders. Antioxidants found in non-starch vegetables help combat inflammation by neutralizing free radicals and inhibiting pro-inflammatory pathways, thereby reducing the risk of chronic inflammation and associated health conditions.

5. **Support Eye Health**: Certain antioxidants found in non-starch vegetables, such as lutein, zeaxanthin, and beta-carotene, are particularly beneficial for eye health.

These antioxidants help protect against age-related macular degeneration, cataracts, and other vision-related issues by filtering harmful blue light and reducing oxidative damage to the eyes.

6. **Protect Cardiovascular Health**: Antioxidants in non-starch vegetables, such as flavonoids and polyphenols, help protect against cardiovascular disease by reducing oxidative stress, lowering inflammation, and improving blood vessel function. Including antioxidant-rich vegetables in the diet can help lower blood pressure, improve cholesterol levels, and reduce the risk of heart disease.

3.4 Weight Management and Digestive Health

Non-starch vegetables play a key role in weight management and digestive health due to their low calorie and high fiber content. Here's how non-starch vegetables support weight management and digestive health:

1. **Low in Calories**: Non-starch vegetables are naturally low in calories and provide bulk to meals without adding significant calories. This makes them ideal for weight management, as they help increase satiety and reduce overall calorie intake without compromising nutritional value.

2. **High in Fiber**: Non-starch vegetables are rich in dietary fiber, which promotes feelings of fullness, aids in digestion, and supports regular bowel movements. Fiber adds bulk to stool, preventing constipation and promoting healthy gut function. Additionally, fiber slows down the absorption of carbohydrates, helping stabilize blood sugar levels and reducing cravings for high-calorie, processed foods.

3. **Hydration**: Many non-starch vegetables, such as cucumbers, tomatoes, and lettuce, have high water content, which contributes to hydration and helps maintain optimal fluid balance in the body. Staying hydrated is essential for proper digestion, nutrient absorption, and overall health.

4. **Gut Health**: The fiber in non-starch vegetables acts as a prebiotic, feeding beneficial bacteria in the gut and promoting a healthy gut microbiome. A balanced gut microbiome is associated with improved digestion, enhanced immune function, and reduced inflammation. Including a variety of fiber-rich vegetables in the diet can help support gut health and digestive function.

5. **Blood Sugar Regulation**: The fiber and water content in non-starch vegetables help slow down the absorption of sugars from carbohydrates, preventing spikes in

blood sugar levels and promoting stable energy levels. This is beneficial for weight management, as well as reducing the risk of type 2 diabetes and metabolic syndrome.

6. **Nutrient Density**: Non-starch vegetables are packed with essential vitamins, minerals, and phytonutrients that support overall health and well-being. By incorporating a variety of vegetables into meals, you can ensure adequate nutrient intake while promoting weight management and digestive health.

non-starch vegetables are valuable components of a balanced diet, offering numerous health benefits related to weight management and digestive health. Including a variety of colorful vegetables in your meals can help support satiety, promote regular bowel movements, and optimize overall health and well-being.

CHAPTER 4

Culinary Uses of Non-Starch Vegetables

4.1 Cooking Methods

Non-starch vegetables are incredibly versatile ingredients that can be prepared using various cooking methods, each imparting unique flavors and textures to dishes. Here are some common cooking methods for non-starch vegetables:

1. **Steaming**: Steaming is a gentle cooking method that helps preserve the nutrients and natural flavors of vegetables. To steam vegetables, place them in a steamer basket or colander over boiling water and cover with a lid. Steam until the vegetables are tender but still crisp, usually for 3 to 5 minutes depending on the vegetable's thickness.

2. **Boiling**: Boiling is a quick and easy way to cook vegetables, although it may result in some nutrient loss due to water-soluble vitamins leaching into the cooking water. To boil vegetables, submerge them in a pot of boiling water and cook until tender. Drain the vegetables and season as desired.

3. **Roasting**: Roasting vegetables in the oven enhances their natural sweetness and caramelizes their sugars, resulting in rich, complex flavors. To roast vegetables, toss them with olive oil, salt, and spices, then spread them out on a baking sheet. Roast in a preheated oven at around 400°F (200°C) until golden brown and tender, stirring occasionally for even cooking.

4. **Sautéing**: Sautéing involves cooking vegetables quickly in a small amount of oil or butter over medium-high heat. This method allows vegetables to develop a golden-brown exterior while retaining their crisp texture. To

sauté vegetables, heat oil or butter in a skillet, add the vegetables, and cook until tender, stirring frequently.

5. **Grilling**: Grilling vegetables adds a smoky flavor and charred exterior, making them perfect for summer cookouts and barbecues. To grill vegetables, brush them with oil and seasonings, then place them directly on a preheated grill over medium-high heat. Cook until tender and slightly charred, turning occasionally for even cooking.

6. **Stir-frying**: Stir-frying is a fast and flavorful cooking method that involves cooking vegetables in a hot pan or wok with a small amount of oil over high heat. This technique preserves the vegetables' crisp texture and vibrant colors. To stir-fry vegetables, heat oil in a wok or skillet, add the vegetables, and cook until tender-crisp, stirring constantly.

7. **Blanching**: Blanching involves briefly boiling vegetables in water,

then immediately plunging them into ice water to stop the cooking process. This method helps retain the vegetables' vibrant colors and crisp texture while partially cooking them. Blanching is often used as a pre-cooking step before freezing vegetables or for preparing vegetables for salads or crudité platters.

8. **Raw**: Some non-starch vegetables can be enjoyed raw, either on their own or as part of salads, sandwiches, wraps, or crudité platters. Raw vegetables provide a crunchy texture and fresh, vibrant flavors, making them a refreshing addition to meals and snacks.

Utilizing these cooking methods, you can unlock the full potential of non-starch vegetables, creating delicious and nutritious dishes that showcase their natural flavors and textures. Experiment with different cooking techniques to discover new ways to enjoy your favorite vegetables and incorporate more plant-based foods into your diet.

4.2 Incorporating Non-Starch Vegetables into Recipes

Non-starch vegetables can be incorporated into a wide range of recipes, adding flavor, texture, and nutritional value to dishes. Here are some creative ways to include non-starch vegetables in your recipes:

1. **Salads**: Create vibrant salads by combining leafy greens with a variety of chopped vegetables such as tomatoes, cucumbers, bell peppers, carrots, and radishes. Add protein sources like grilled chicken, tofu, or chickpeas for a satisfying meal.

2. **Stir-fries and Stir-fry Bowls**: Stir-fries are versatile dishes that allow you to showcase a variety of vegetables. Stir-fry colorful

vegetables like broccoli, bell peppers, snap peas, and mushrooms with protein sources like tofu, shrimp, or beef, and serve over rice or noodles for a quick and nutritious meal.

3. **Soups and Stews**: Add depth and flavor to soups and stews by incorporating non-starch vegetables such as onions, carrots, celery, tomatoes, and spinach. Use vegetable broth as a base and experiment with different herbs and spices to enhance the taste.

4. **Roasted Vegetable Medleys**: Create delicious roasted vegetable medleys by tossing chopped vegetables like potatoes, carrots, cauliflower, and Brussels sprouts with olive oil, salt, and spices. Roast in the oven until caramelized and tender for a flavorful side dish or main course.

5. **Vegetable Pasta Dishes**: Incorporate non-starch vegetables into pasta dishes by adding sautéed or roasted

vegetables to pasta sauces or tossing them with cooked pasta. Try combinations like spaghetti with cherry tomatoes and basil, or penne with spinach, mushrooms, and garlic.

6. **Vegetable Frittatas and Quiches**: Make vegetable-packed frittatas and quiches by mixing sautéed vegetables such as onions, peppers, spinach, and zucchini with eggs and cheese. Bake until set for a nutritious breakfast, brunch, or dinner option.

7. **Vegetable Wraps and Rolls**: Use large lettuce leaves or collard greens as wraps for filling them with a variety of vegetables, protein, and condiments. Fill wraps with ingredients like grilled vegetables, avocado, hummus, and grilled chicken for a healthy and portable meal.

8. **Grilled Vegetable Skewers**: Thread chunks of vegetables like bell peppers, zucchini, cherry tomatoes, and mushrooms onto skewers and

grill until tender and lightly charred. Serve as a colorful and flavorful side dish or appetizer.

Incorporating non-starch vegetables into your recipes, you can add nutritional value, color, and flavor to your meals while enjoying the health benefits of these versatile ingredients.

4.3 Raw vs. Cooked Non-Starch Vegetables

Both raw and cooked non-starch vegetables offer unique benefits and flavors, and incorporating a variety of both into your diet can provide optimal nutrition. Here's a comparison between raw and cooked non-starch vegetables:

Raw Non-Starch Vegetables:

1. **Nutrient Retention**: Raw vegetables retain more of their vitamins and minerals compared to cooked vegetables, as heat can degrade

certain nutrients like vitamin C and folate.

2. **Crunch and Texture**: Raw vegetables provide a crisp texture and crunchiness that can add freshness and vibrancy to salads, wraps, and snacks.

3. **Hydration**: Raw vegetables have a high-water content, which can help hydrate the body and contribute to feelings of fullness and satiety.

4. **Digestive Enzymes**: Raw vegetables contain natural enzymes that aid in digestion and may support gut health and nutrient absorption.

5. **Convenience**: Raw vegetables require minimal preparation and can be enjoyed on the go as snacks or added to salads and sandwiches for quick and easy meals.

Cooked Non-Starch Vegetables:

1. **Enhanced Flavor**: Cooking can enhance the natural sweetness and

flavors of vegetables, making them
more palatable and enjoyable for
some individuals.

2. **Improved Digestibility**: Cooking
    breaks down tough fibers and cell
    walls in vegetables, making them
    easier to digest and absorb nutrients.

3. **Versatility**: Cooked vegetables can
    be incorporated into a wide range of
    dishes, including soups, stir-fries,
    casseroles, and pasta dishes,
    allowing for greater culinary
    creativity and variety.

4. **Increased Antioxidant
    Availability**: While some nutrients
    may be lost during cooking, certain
    cooking methods can increase the
    availability of antioxidants and other
    beneficial compounds in vegetables.

5. **Longer Shelf Life**: Cooking can
    extend the shelf life of vegetables by
    slowing down spoilage and microbial
    growth, allowing for greater

flexibility in meal planning and preparation.

Both raw and cooked non-starch vegetables into your diet allows you to enjoy a diverse array of flavors, textures, and nutritional benefits. Experiment with different cooking methods and preparation techniques to discover your favorite ways to enjoy these nutritious ingredients.

CHAPTER 5

Selecting and Storing Non-Starch Vegetables

5.1 Choosing Fresh Non-Starch Vegetables

Selecting fresh non-starch vegetables is essential to ensure optimal flavor, texture, and nutritional quality. Here are some tips for choosing the best non-starch vegetables at the grocery store or farmers' market:

1. **Appearance**: Look for non-starch vegetables that are vibrant in color, with firm, crisp textures. Avoid vegetables that appear wilted, discolored, or have soft spots, as these may indicate spoilage or dehydration.

2. **Texture**: Choose vegetables that feel heavy for their size and have smooth, unblemished skin. Avoid vegetables

with wrinkled or shriveled skin, as this may indicate dehydration or loss of freshness.

3. **Smell**: Some vegetables, such as onions and garlic, may have a mild aroma that indicates freshness. However, strong or unpleasant odors can be a sign of spoilage or decay, so avoid vegetables with off-putting smells.

4. **Seasonality**: Whenever possible, choose non-starch vegetables that are in season, as they are likely to be fresher, tastier, and more affordable. Seasonal vegetables also tend to have higher nutritional content and better flavor compared to out-of-season produce.

5. **Organic Options**: Consider purchasing organic non-starch vegetables, especially for varieties that are known to have higher pesticide residues. Organic produce is grown without synthetic pesticides and fertilizers, which may be

beneficial for both human health and the environment.

6. **Local Produce**: Support local farmers by choosing locally grown non-starch vegetables when available. Locally sourced produce is often fresher, tastier, and more environmentally sustainable than imported varieties, as it requires less transportation and storage.

5.2 Storing Fresh Non-Starch Vegetables

Proper storage helps preserve the freshness and quality of non-starch vegetables, extending their shelf life and minimizing food waste. Here are some general guidelines for storing fresh non-starch vegetables:

1. **Refrigeration**: Most non-starch vegetables should be stored in the refrigerator to maintain freshness. Place vegetables in the crisper

drawer or in perforated plastic bags to help retain moisture and prevent wilting.

2. **Separation**: Store different types of vegetables separately to prevent them from affecting each other's flavor and ripening process. Some vegetables, like tomatoes and bananas, release ethylene gas, which can accelerate the ripening of other produce.

3. **Moisture Control**: Some vegetables, such as leafy greens and herbs, benefit from slightly damp conditions to prevent wilting. Wrap these vegetables in damp paper towels or store them in breathable produce bags to maintain moisture levels.

4. **Air Circulation**: Ensure proper air circulation in the refrigerator to prevent moisture buildup and reduce the risk of mold and spoilage. Avoid overcrowding the refrigerator and

leave space between items for air to circulate freely.

5. **Temperature**: Keep the refrigerator temperature set between 35°F to 40°F (1.7°C to 4.4°C) to slow down the ripening process and extend the shelf life of non-starch vegetables. Use a refrigerator thermometer to monitor and adjust the temperature as needed.

6. **Use in a Timely Manner**: Fresh non-starch vegetables have a limited shelf life and should be consumed within a few days to a week of purchase for optimal flavor and nutritional quality. Plan meals accordingly to use up perishable vegetables before they spoil.

7. **Root Vegetables**: Root vegetables like potatoes, carrots, and beets should be stored in a cool, dark, and well-ventilated place, such as a pantry or cellar. Avoid storing them in plastic bags, as this can trap moisture and promote rotting.

8. **Herbs**: Fresh herbs can be stored like bouquets of flowers by placing them in a glass of water and covering the leaves loosely with a plastic bag. Alternatively, wrap herbs in damp paper towels and store them in a resealable plastic bag in the refrigerator.

9. **Ethylene-sensitive Vegetables**: Some vegetables, such as broccoli, cauliflower, and asparagus, are sensitive to ethylene gas and should be stored separately from ethylene-producing fruits like apples and bananas to prevent premature ripening and spoilage.

10. **Check and Rotate**: Regularly check the condition of stored vegetables and discard any that show signs of spoilage or decay. Use older vegetables before fresher ones to minimize food waste and ensure optimal quality.

These proper storage techniques, you can prolong the shelf life of non-starch vegetables and enjoy fresh, flavorful produce for longer periods, minimizing waste and maximizing nutritional benefits.

5.3 Tips for Maximizing Freshness and Flavor

Maximizing the freshness and flavor of non-starch vegetables requires attention to detail from the moment of purchase to the time of consumption. Here are some tips to help you get the most out of your vegetables:

1. **Buy Seasonal and Local**: Opt for seasonal and locally grown non-starch vegetables whenever possible. They are likely to be fresher, tastier, and more nutritious than out-of-season or imported varieties.

2. **Inspect Carefully**: When selecting vegetables at the store or market, carefully inspect them for signs of freshness. Look for vibrant colors, firm textures, and no signs of wilting, browning, or bruising.

3. **Shop Often**: Purchase smaller quantities of non-starch vegetables more frequently to ensure you're using them at the peak of freshness. This also helps minimize waste and ensures you have a variety of fresh options on hand.

4. **Store Properly**: Follow proper storage techniques, such as refrigeration, temperature control, and separation, to maintain the freshness of your vegetables and extend their shelf life.

5. **Handle with Care**: Handle non-starch vegetables gently to avoid bruising or damage, which can accelerate spoilage. Avoid squeezing or crushing delicate vegetables and use a sharp knife to minimize cell damage.

6. **Clean Thoroughly**: Wash non-starch vegetables under cold, running water before consuming or cooking them to remove dirt, bacteria, and pesticide residues. Use a vegetable

brush for firm-skinned vegetables and leafy greens.

7. **Trim and Prepare Fresh**: Trim any wilted or damaged parts from vegetables before storing or using them. Prepare vegetables just before cooking or serving to preserve their texture, flavor, and nutritional content.

8. **Use the Whole Vegetable**: Whenever possible, use the entire vegetable, including stems, leaves, and peels, to minimize waste and maximize nutritional value. Many vegetable parts are edible and nutritious.

9. **Enhance with Herbs and Spices**: Boost the flavor of non-starch vegetables by seasoning them with herbs, spices, garlic, onions, citrus zest, or vinegar. Experiment with different flavor combinations to create delicious and satisfying dishes.

10. **Cook with Care**: Choose cooking methods that preserve the natural flavors and textures of vegetables, such as steaming, roasting, grilling, or sautéing. Avoid overcooking vegetables, as this can result in loss of flavor and nutrients.

11. **Pair Thoughtfully**: Combine non-starch vegetables with complementary ingredients to enhance their flavor and nutritional value. Incorporate a variety of vegetables into meals to create balanced and flavorful dishes.

12. **Store Cut Vegetables Properly**: If you've cut vegetables in advance, store them in an airtight container in the refrigerator to prevent them from drying out or absorbing odors. Use them within a few days for best results.

CHAPTER 6

Risks and Considerations

6.1 Potential Allergies or Sensitivities

Potential allergies or sensitivities to non-starch vegetables are relatively rare compared to other food allergies, but they can still occur. Here are some considerations regarding allergies or sensitivities to non-starch vegetables:

1. **Common Allergies**: While uncommon, some individuals may have allergies to specific non-starch vegetables, such as certain varieties of nightshades (e.g., tomatoes, eggplants, peppers), cruciferous vegetables (e.g., broccoli, cabbage, Brussels sprouts), or allium vegetables (e.g., onions, garlic, leeks). Allergic reactions can range from mild symptoms like itching,

swelling, or hives to more severe reactions such as difficulty breathing or anaphylaxis.

2. **Cross-reactivity**: Individuals with allergies to certain pollens may experience oral allergy syndrome (OAS) when consuming certain raw fruits or vegetables. For example, those allergic to birch pollen may experience symptoms when eating raw fruits and vegetables like apples, cherries, carrots, and celery due to cross-reactivity. Cooking the vegetables may eliminate this reaction for some individuals.

3. **Latex-Fruit Syndrome**: Some individuals allergic to latex may also experience allergic reactions to certain fruits and vegetables due to cross-reactivity. This condition, known as latex-fruit syndrome, can cause symptoms such as itching, swelling, or hives when consuming fruits and vegetables such as bananas, avocados, kiwis, and chestnuts.

4. **Histamine Intolerance**: Non-starch vegetables, particularly those that are aged, fermented, or high in histamine content (such as tomatoes, spinach, and eggplant), may trigger symptoms in individuals with histamine intolerance. Symptoms can include headaches, migraines, digestive issues, and skin reactions.

5. **Food Sensitivities**: Some individuals may experience sensitivities rather than true allergies to certain non-starch vegetables. Sensitivities can manifest as gastrointestinal discomfort, bloating, gas, or other digestive symptoms after consuming certain vegetables. Identifying and eliminating trigger foods through an elimination diet or food journaling can help manage sensitivities.

6. **Precautions**: If you suspect an allergy or sensitivity to non-starch vegetables, consult with a healthcare professional for proper diagnosis and management. Allergy testing, dietary adjustments, and avoidance of

trigger foods may be recommended depending on the severity of the reaction.

7. **Cooking Methods**: Cooking vegetables can sometimes alter their allergenic properties or reduce the likelihood of triggering allergic reactions. For example, individuals with pollen allergies may tolerate cooked vegetables better than raw ones due to changes in protein structures during cooking.

8. **Reading Labels**: Individuals with known allergies or sensitivities should carefully read food labels and ask about ingredient information when dining out to avoid potential allergens or cross-contamination.

While allergies or sensitivities to non-starch vegetables are relatively uncommon, it's essential to be aware of potential risks and considerations, especially for individuals with known food allergies or sensitivities. Consulting with a healthcare professional or allergist can provide personalized guidance and recommendations for managing allergies or sensitivities to non-starch vegetables.

6.2 Pesticide Residue and Organic Options

Pesticide residue is a concern associated with conventionally grown non-starch vegetables, as pesticides are commonly used in agriculture to control pests and diseases. Here are some considerations regarding pesticide residue and organic options:

1. **Pesticide Use**: Conventionally grown non-starch vegetables may contain pesticide residues from the application of synthetic pesticides during cultivation. Pesticide residues can remain on the surface of vegetables, even after washing, and may pose health risks if consumed in high quantities over time.

2. **Health Concerns**: Exposure to pesticide residues has been linked to

various health concerns, including an increased risk of certain cancers, hormone disruption, reproductive issues, neurodevelopmental disorders, and adverse effects on the immune system. Children, pregnant women, and individuals with compromised immune systems may be more susceptible to the adverse effects of pesticide exposure.

3. **Organic Certification**: Organic farming practices prohibit the use of synthetic pesticides, herbicides, and fertilizers. Instead, organic farmers use natural methods such as crop rotation, biological pest control, and organic-approved pesticides to manage pests and diseases. Organic certification ensures that the produce has been grown and processed according to strict organic standards set by certifying bodies.

4. **Benefits of Organic**: Choosing organic non-starch vegetables can reduce exposure to pesticide residues and synthetic chemicals, promoting

environmental sustainability and supporting soil health. Organic farming practices also prioritize biodiversity, conservation of natural resources, and the reduction of pollution and environmental degradation.

5. **Cost Considerations**: Organic non-starch vegetables may be more expensive than their conventionally grown counterparts due to higher production costs, certification requirements, and lower yields associated with organic farming practices. However, some consumers prioritize the health and environmental benefits of organic produce and are willing to pay a premium for certified organic options.

6. **Washing and Peeling**: Washing non-starch vegetables thoroughly under running water and peeling certain vegetables can help reduce pesticide residues on the surface. However, peeling may also remove

some nutrients and beneficial compounds found in the skin, so it's essential to weigh the potential benefits and drawbacks.

7. **Supporting Local Farmers**: Buying directly from local farmers or participating in community-supported agriculture (CSA) programs can provide access to freshly harvested, sustainably grown non-starch vegetables. Many small-scale farmers follow organic or low-input farming practices, even if they are not certified organic.

8. **Certification Labels**: Look for certification labels such as USDA Organic, EU Organic, or other recognized organic certification logos when purchasing organic non-starch vegetables. These labels indicate that the produce meets specific organic standards and has been certified by a reputable certifying body.

Overall, choosing organic non-starch vegetables can help reduce exposure to pesticide residues and support sustainable agricultural practices. However, it's essential to consider individual preferences, budget constraints, and availability when making purchasing decisions. Washing, peeling, and supporting local farmers are additional strategies to minimize pesticide exposure and promote health and environmental sustainability.

CHAPTER 7

Encouraging Non-Starch Vegetable Consumption

Encouraging non-starch vegetable consumption is crucial for promoting overall health and well-being, as these nutrient-dense foods offer numerous health benefits. Here are some strategies for promoting the consumption of non-starch vegetables:

1. **Lead by Example**: Set a positive example by incorporating non-starch vegetables into your own meals and snacks. Show enthusiasm for trying new vegetables and experimenting with different cooking methods and recipes.

2. **Educate About Benefits**: Educate others about the health benefits of non-starch vegetables, including their high nutrient content, fiber, antioxidants, and potential to reduce

the risk of chronic diseases such as heart disease, diabetes, and certain types of cancer.

3. **Make Vegetables Visible and Accessible**: Keep a variety of fresh non-starch vegetables readily available and visible in your kitchen. Store pre-cut vegetables in clear containers at eye level in the refrigerator for easy access and quick snacks.

4. **Incorporate Into Meals**: Find creative ways to incorporate non-starch vegetables into meals and snacks. Add vegetables to omelets, stir-fries, soups, salads, sandwiches, wraps, smoothies, and pasta dishes for added flavor, texture, and nutrition.

5. **Experiment with Flavors and Textures**: Encourage trying different types of non-starch vegetables and experimenting with various flavors and textures. Roast vegetables with herbs and spices, grill them for a

smoky flavor, or enjoy them raw
with dips and dressings for a crunchy
snack.

6. **Get Children Involved**: Involve
children in meal planning, grocery
shopping, and food preparation to
increase their interest and excitement
about non-starch vegetables. Let
them choose vegetables to try and
explore new recipes together as a
family.

7. **Add Variety to Meals**: Offer a
variety of non-starch vegetables in
different colors, shapes, and textures
to make meals more visually
appealing and enjoyable. Incorporate
a rainbow of vegetables to ensure a
diverse range of nutrients and
flavors.

8. **Offer Tasty Dips and Sauces**: Serve
non-starch vegetables with tasty dips
and sauces to enhance their flavor
and appeal. Hummus, guacamole,
salsa, tzatziki, peanut sauce, and
tahini dressing are delicious options

that pair well with raw or cooked
vegetables.

9. **Celebrate Seasonal Produce**:
    Embrace seasonal eating by
    highlighting fresh, locally grown
    non-starch vegetables in your meals.
    Visit farmers' markets or participate
    in community-supported agriculture
    (CSA) programs to access a variety
    of seasonal produce.

10. **Provide Positive Reinforcement**:
    Praise and encourage individuals for
    choosing and enjoying non-starch
    vegetables. Celebrate small victories
    and accomplishments related to
    vegetable consumption to reinforce
    healthy eating habits.

11. **Be Patient and Persistent**: Be
    patient and persistent when
    introducing non-starch vegetables to
    picky eaters or individuals who are
    hesitant to try new foods. Offer
    vegetables in different forms and
    preparations, and give individuals

time to adjust to new flavors and textures.

By implementing these strategies, you can help encourage and promote the consumption of non-starch vegetables among individuals of all ages, fostering healthier eating habits and improving overall dietary quality.

www.ingramcontent.com/pod-product-compliance
Lightning Source LLC
Chambersburg PA
CBHW050825250726
48653CB00006B/2421